Parkinson's:

Common

Threads

A comparative survey.

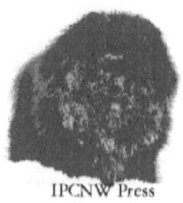

IPCNW Press

Parkinson's Database Survey is a Registered
Copyright

©TXu 1-847-332

www.parkinsonsdatabase.com

A Note from the Author

In July of 2011 I was diagnosed with idiopathic Parkinson's disease at the age of 41. With the diagnosis I immediately began to research the causes and many facets of the disease. I found it a little disturbing that there were literally no answers from the doctors as to what had caused it. Even more bothersome was the fact that once diagnosed there was no longer an urgency or for that matter an interest in what the cause was. It felt like game over as I persisted in pressuring doctors of many specialties to continue testing, much of which was turned down or flatly dismissed.

As I researched the disease, I found that there were in fact many possible and even probable known causes. Why wouldn't they investigate? Why was there no longer a need to understand what was really going on? I was told time and time again that "we just don't know", along with "I hear that all the time". This just wasn't good enough for me and shouldn't be for anyone.

I discovered that there was in fact a great deal known about Parkinson's, enough to fill a University library. So why was there such an aura of mystery surrounding the disease? I realized that most of the information came from studies involving rats that were deliberately given Parkinson's, many times introduced directly into the brain. This is obviously not how Parkinson's develops and humans are in fact not rats, there are certainly differences.

I wondered what the common threads were amongst Parkinson's patients. During my research I found thousands of studies, most of which claimed to have found a breakthrough in research. I quickly focused on the percentages in the studies and found that a "breakthrough" often meant that 1-3% of study participants exhibited particular symptoms or met certain criteria. Unfortunately, all of these low percentage breakthroughs are not a breakthrough of any kind, they coincide with the total population and the incidence of Parkinson's and reveal nothing of value.

I decided that anything with a percentage basis of 5% or less was baseless, 10% or less was probably irrelevant but worth looking into, 15% was of interest, 20% was absolutely worthy of further investigation and anything over 30% was probably definitive. One of the things I noticed was absent was input from patients and people actually living with the disease, such as myself. Why would we not have detailed information obtained from patients compiled into some type of database to help point researchers in the right direction? What could be more valuable for research?

In 2013 the Parkinson's Database Survey© was launched as a means to create a comparative analysis of some of the many aspects of the average Parkinson's patient's life and condition. No personally identifiable information was collected for the survey other than Zip code. The results are randomized and anonymous.

The survey contains seven sections with a total of 115 different questions for Parkinson's patients with the intent to solidify much of what is already known about Parkinson's, separate some of the myth from fact as well as finding common associations in the disease that are perhaps overlooked or miscalculated.

There were a total of 2302 responses of which 2218 were disqualified due to incompleteness or other factors that might affect the validity of the data. The disqualified responses were collected in a sample survey which contained clear notations that the responses would not be considered. 84 complete responses were considered and reviewed for this text to keep the margin of error extremely minimal. The surveys were completed blindly as no results have ever been released prior to this work.

The survey remains open and anonymous. There are two options for taking the survey. The full survey can be completed with a simple registration, or it can be taken in 7 parts divided by category.

The data in this book is presented in 7 different sections, each of which correlates to one section of the survey. Each question is listed individually. Some are followed by a short commentary relating to the response ratio, the significance of the question and my personal opinions on not only Parkinson's but also some of the politics and failures that hinder or inhibit research.

The responses are shown in percentages only for ease of use. Inline data was withheld as this book is simply meant to present straight forward data to either corroborate or dismiss some of the many theories related to Parkinson's disease.

If you have Parkinson's, I highly recommend that you complete the survey or take any portion of the survey that you feel is relevant. Information from patients is critical in understanding this disease and its many different etiologies. It is completely anonymous and we never ask for any type of personal information, or contributions of any kind.

I sincerely hope that you find the information useful and that it provides at least a little insight into what may or may not have caused yours or a family member's illness. If it gives researchers insight or direction that will help the Parkinson's community then I have succeeded in doing my part. At least for now.

As patients, we need to help drive awareness and understanding of Parkinson's disease. The lack of understanding by others is one of the biggest hurdles in living with this illness. It is not anyone's fault for not understanding. As most if not all of us know, it is extremely difficult to explain what is going on physically. It is almost something that cannot be understood without experiencing it. Learning to share what is happening without overwhelming people comes in time. Be patient and thoughtful with those around you, they will understand.

Live your life to the fullest and accept what you have been given. Things we be alright, they always are.

Steven

General Questions

1) Is this form being competed with assistance?

Yes 7.14%

No 71.43%

This data coincides with the inference that a majority of patients are physically and cognitively able to understand and complete information related to their current lifestyle, physical condition, and history. It also corroborates the belief that most patients are functional able to complete regular tasks as would any other person. This is entirely expected and probably why Parkinson's is sometimes considered a minor ailment.

2) Have you or the person you are completing this form for been diagnosed with Parkinson's?

Yes 78.57%

No 0.00%

3) Select the Neurological syndrome you have been diagnosed with.

No patients completing this survey listed any other neurological condition other than Parkinson's as a diagnosis.

4) Is the diagnosis 'Idiopathic' or without known cause?

Yes 72.62%

No 4.76%

With so many cases being diagnosed as idiopathic, it is critical to make distinctions between the different variations of the disease. This is a key areas of research that must be pursued. Having no known cause with such a large population of patients makes research exceedingly difficult on nearly any level. More focus certainly needs to be placed on the root cause as well as symptomatic treatment. Isolating specific causes will expedite the path to finding a cure and better symptomatic treatment. A majority of Parkinson's cases fall into this category.

5) What is your total UPDRS score for parts I, II & III? (If known)

6) What is your total UPDRS score for parts IV & V? (If known)

Astonishingly only 3 patients of the 84 were aware of the UPDRS score for parts I, II & III and only 2 patients were aware of their score for parts IV & V. I was a part of the group that was never given this information. It truly felt like deception once I realized that all of the seemingly furious note taking by the neurologist was actually a rating scale that I would never see. The scale is owned and licensed by the International Parkinson and Movement Disorder Society. This should not be a scale used for financial gain, nor should it be withheld from patients.

This indicates that there is likely a major defect in the lines of communication between doctors and patients. It is terribly important that the patient understand the physicians' position and projected course of treatment, as well as clearly communicating every aspect of their condition. There should be no information that should not be disseminated from doctor to patient or vice versa at any time. All patients should know their UPDRS score and what it means. This is a responsibility that falls squarely on the shoulders of the physician.

3

7) Are you incapacitated?

Not at all 34.52%

Somewhat 27.38%

Partially 13.10%

Completely3.57%

It is well known that a majority of Parkinson's patients are capable of functioning on some level. This is most likely due to the fact that there is symptomatic treatment that is at least somewhat effective. On a different level it may also indicate a lack of resources or available options for patients as they progress through the disease. Many have no alternative other than to continue working while struggling with the illness. Parkinson's patients become experts at hiding their symptoms and many continue to work and lead productive lives. Disability levels should be assessed and evaluated regularly both to monitor and continue treatment and ensure that the patient has access to proper accommodations when necessary.

8) Are you able to work?

Not at all   22.62%

    0-10 Hours per week   10.71%

10-20 Hours per week   8.33%

20-30 Hours per week   5.95%

30-40 Hours per week   17.86%

More than 40 Hours   13.10%

It can be inferred from questions 7 and 8 that nearly 45% of patients have work limitations of 30 hours or less. This correlates almost directly to the 44% of those stating that there is some type of incapacity at play rather than none at all. This is assuming that the lesser work hours are related to the incapacitation and not economic factors.

9) Do you require assistance or a care giver?

Yes 19.05%

No 59.52%

Most patients live for many years without the need of a caregiver. There are daily struggles but they are often overcome with patience and diligence. As with any disability, most tend to find ways to cope with the impairments as much as possible. It really is important for patients to try to stay active and do for themselves, especially from an emotional standpoint. In any type of chronic illness, it can be easy to lose purpose.

10) Please indicate which activities require assistance.

Bathing	10.71%
Communicating	7.14%
Cooking	9.52%
Dressing	8.33%
Driving	11.90%
Personal Hygiene	5.95%
Walking	8.33%

This question is linked to the previous and would only prompt with a "Yes" answer to requiring the assistance of a caregiver.

11) Is your condition painful?

Yes 36.90%

No 41.67%

12) What part of your body hurts?

Head   7.14%

Neck   25.00%

Shoulders 27.38%

Chest   2.38%

Abdomen 2.38%

Pelvis   3.57%

Middle Back 11.90%

Sides of back   8.33%

Upper arm   9.52%

Lower arm 10.71%

Hands   13.10%

Lower back 17.86%

Hips   11.90%

Buttocks   3.57%

Thighs (front) 3.57%

Thighs (back) 5.95%

Knees	11.90%
Calves	14.29%
Ankles	7.14%
Feet	21.43%

13) Please indicate if your pain is aching in the appropriate boxes.

Head 7.14%

Neck 22.62%

Shoulders 22.62%

Chest 1.19%

Abdomen 2.38%

Pelvis 1.19%

Middle Back 8.33%

Sides of back 7.14%

Upper arm 9.52%

Lower arm 7.14%

Hands 5.95%

Lower back 10.71%

Hips 8.33%

Buttocks 3.57%

Thighs (front) 4.76%

Thighs (back) 5.95%

Knees 11.90%

Calves 9.52%

Ankles 4.76%

Feet 16.67%

14) Please indicate if your pain is stabbing or piercing in the appropriate boxes.

Head 3.57%

Neck 8.33%

Shoulders 4.76%

Chest 1.19%

Abdomen 2.38%

Pelvis 0.00%

Middle Back 3.57%

Sides of back 2.38%

Upper arm 1.19%

Lower arm 1.19%

Hands 3.57%

Lower back 7.14%

Hips 3.57%

Buttocks 1.19%

Thighs (front) 0.00%

Thighs (back) 0.00%

Knees 2.38%

Calves 2.38%

Ankles 2.38%

Feet 5.95%

None 13.10%

It can be clearly seen that Parkinson's disease is a painful condition for many. It is interesting to note that the pain reported is primarily that of the aching type. Much of that pain is centered in the neck and shoulder areas followed by the feet. More than 20% of the respondents indicated pain in each of these areas. It is also significant that the percentage that identified it as aching pain rather than sharp or piercing pain was considerably higher. The reasons for this certainly merit further study and investigation. Is there anything being overlooked?

15) Are your symptoms consistent from day to day?

Yes 48.81%

No 29.76%

Two things that are known to affect symptoms on a daily basis are sleep patterns and dietary intake. Protein is known to affect levodopa absorption and can be a factor. Sound sleep can also lead to a reduction in the intensity of symptoms on a daily basis.

16) Do you get relief from your symptoms by resting? (Even if temporary)

Yes 59.52%

No 19.05%

17) Are your symptoms present when you run or perform other vigorous physical activities?

Yes 55.95%

No 21.43%

It is not understood why periods of rest are helpful but there is a definite majority that benefit from rest. Understanding whether this is simply muscular relief or if it is related to serotonin, cortisol and melatonin production would yield valuable clues to this mystery and could provide better pathways to treatment.

Many patients benefit from exercise. Again, it is not fully understood why. Curiously, some report being completely free of symptoms when exercising or doing other rigorous physical activities but this appears to be the exception rather than the norm. Types of exercise and how it each affects specific symptoms should be closely studied and evaluated. This could provide better guidelines for prescribing therapy in the different etiologies of the disease.

Demographics

18) What is your age?

An average age of 59 was recorded with the lowest being 37 and the highest of 89.

19) At what age were you diagnosed?

The average age of diagnosis is 54 with the lowest being 32 and the highest of 87.

20) What is your gender?

Female40.48%

Male34.52%

This is interesting because it is often noted that men are more prone to Parkinson's than women. Perhaps it is just an indication that women are more likely to take an active approach to understanding and coping with the condition.

21) What is your height?

22) What is your weight?

Height ranges were 5′1″ to 6′5″. Weight ranges were from 84 lbs. to 295 lbs. This indicates that BMI is probably not a factor in Parkinson's disease.

23) What do you consider your ethnicity?

African American	1.19%
American Indian	1.19%
Caucasian	53.57%
Celtic	8.33%
Czech	2.38%
English	16.67%
Finnish	1.19%
French	5.95%
German	9.52%

Hispanic or Latino   1.19%

Italian   1.19%

Latvian   1.19%

Middle Eastern   2.38%

Polish   2.38%

Russian   1.19%

Scandinavian   3.57%

Scottish   2.38%

Spanish (Europe) 4.76%

Swedish   1.19%

24) What is your eye color?

Amber   0.00%

Blue 22.62%

Brown 26.19%

Gray   4.76%

Green 11.90%

Hazel   8.33%

25) What is your hair color?

Auburn hair   3.57%

Black hair   4.76%

Blond hair   9.52%

Brown hair   30.95%

Chestnut hair   0.00%

Red hair   2.38%

Gray and white hair 19.05%

Although Caucasians appear to be more likely to get Parkinson's, there is no indication that hair color or eye color bear any relevance. It should be noted that those of English descent have an incidence much higher than most. This could be an indication of genetic susceptibility as this question asked ethnicity, not location.

26) Have any members of your family been diagnosed with Parkinson's?

Yes 23.81%

No 48.81%

27) Are they a blood relative?

Yes 23.81%

This is consistent with estimates of familial Parkinson's. Strong consideration for environmental causes should be made in familial cases. It may not be who the people are, rather it may where they are that is a factor. There are known geographic clusters of neurological conditions such as ALS and Parkinson's.

28) Do you live in the United States?

Yes 55.95%

No 17.86%

29) Please enter your 5 digit ZIP code.

ZIP codes were somewhat evenly distributed across the United States. There is not enough data to make any accurate assessments.

A simple requirement for physicians to report age, gender and postal code would open new doors in Parkinson's research. In today's world of technology there is no excuse for not having this system in place. It is a political failure as well as a failure on the part of the medical community.

30) Please enter your Country.

Australia 3.57%

Canada 2.38%

France 1.19%

Iran 1.19%

Lithuania 1.19%

Mexico 1.19%

New Zealand 1.19%

Spain 1.19%

United Kingdom 3.57%

United States 83.34%

31) What type of dwelling do you live in?

Apartment 3.57%

Duplex 3.57%

House 63.10%

Mobile Home 3.57%

32) What is the age of your dwelling?

The average dwelling age was 43 years, ranging from 1 years old to 160 years.

This series of questions is to determine if there could be any association between chemicals used in building materials from a particular time period and Parkinson's cases.

The distribution of home age was evenly distributed. 63% of respondents resided in a house, and 32% of those homes had been remodeled, there doesn't appear to be any association with construction materials of a specific time period and Parkinson's disease based on this data.

33) Do you have Gas Appliances?

Yes 41.67%

No 32.14%

34) Do you have a wood burning Stove?

Yes 10.71%

No 63.10%

35) What is your primary heat source?

Coal   0.00%

Gas 39.29%

Electric 22.62%

Oil   5.95%

Other   3.57%

Wood   2.38%

36) Do you cook with Charcoal or Wood?

Yes 4.76%

No 69.05%

Carbon monoxide poisoning in severe cases is known to cause Parkinsonism. This kind of poisoning can often be identified on an MRI as basal ganglia degeneration is often present.

37) Has your home been remodeled?

Yes 32.14%

No 41.67%

38) When was it remodeled?

5 Years ago, 16.67%

10 Years ago, 5.95%

15 Years ago, 7.14%

20 Years ago, 1.19%

More than 20 Years ago 1.19%

39) Has there been construction or drilling in areas that you have lived?

Yes 30.95%

No 42.86%

40) Have you lived on or near a Farm?

Crop Producing 26.19%

Dairy   8.33%

Livestock 16.67%

Mixed 21.43%

None of the above 33.33%

Farming areas are known to have higher incidences of Parkinson's disease. Most indications are that pesticides and herbicides could be responsible for many cases of Parkinson's, crop producing being the highest risk. Crop producing and mixed farming are obviously prevalent here supporting the belief that pesticides and or their derivatives m ay play a key role.

41) What type of water system do you have? (Check all that apply)

Community 7.14%

Municipal 51.19%

Natural Water Source 4.76%

Septic 11.90%

Sewer 11.90%

Well 15.48%

42) Do you have a recent water quality report?

Yes 9.52%

No 63.10%

43) Were any of the following chemicals present?

2,4-D 0.00%

Acrylamide 0.00%

Aluminum 0.00%

Arsenic 2.38%

Barium 1.19%

Cadmium 0.00%

Carbofuran 0.00%

Chlordane 0.00%

Chloride 1.19%

Chlorine 2.38%

Chlorine dioxide 0.00%

Chromium 1.19%

Coliform 2.38%

Copper 3.57%

Cryptosporidium 0.00%

Cyanide 0.00%

Fluoride 2.38%

Glyphosate 0.00%

Haloacetic acids 2.38%

Iron 1.19%

Lead 3.57%

Manganese 1.19%

Mercury 0.00%

Methane 0.00%

Nitrate 3.57%

Organic Carbon 0.00%

Oxamyl 0.00%

PCB's 0.00%

Selenium 1.19%

Sulfate 0.00%

T 1,1,1-Trichloroethaneoluene 0.00%

Trihalomethane 1.19%

Xylenes 0.00%

It is alarming knowing that so few people have copies of their water report. It is an archaic system run by the EPA that lacks the use of current technology to make this data easily accessible and available. What is even more concerning is the fact that many of the chemicals listed above are not typically checked on Consumer Confidence Reports. Additionally, there are many chemicals that can potentially leech in to ground water that are not currently considered to be harmful but are strongly suspected of many types of illness. Industrial solvents are likely the most toxic. Periodically it is discovered that some of these solvents have been seeping into groundwater for years and then it is suddenly and coincidentally discovered that people in those areas are not well. This is an absolute failure of the water quality system which is in dire need of complete revision.

It is entirely reasonable to believe that chemicals in drinking water could have a direct link to neurological problems. Cyanobacteria or blue green algae for example is suspected of causing ALS and other types of neurological problems. It thrives in nutrient rich water such as lakes polluted with phosphates from fertilizer run off. This is just another example of how important it is to ensure that our waters are not tainted by chemicals.

44) Do you live near or have you ever lived near overhead power lines?

Yes 22.62%

No 51.19%

45) Do you have or have you ever had an indoor cat?

Yes 51.19%

No 22.62%

46) Do you clean or have you ever cleaned a litter box?

Yes 50.00%

No 1.19

47) Does your cat sleep with you?

Yes 13.10%

No 38.10%

H. Pylori a bacteria found in cat feces and it is periodically a consideration for Parkinsonism. It is a spirochete and should not be entirely discounted in all cases. This type of infection is usually identifiable through blood tests and symptomatic diagnosis. Spirochete's such as Borrelia burgdorferi (Lyme) and Treponema pallidum (syphilis) can in fact cause neurological problems but are rarely implicated in Parkinson's due to the fact that there are very specific symptoms associated with them, most of which are not present in Parkinson's. Neurological conditions also tend to present in late stages of these diseases after what can be a prolonged latent period. It is also common for the presentation to be bi-lateral in spirochete infections which is not indicative of idiopathic Parkinson's. Nonetheless, accurate blood tests for spirochetes should be completed and ruled out on all patients.

48) Do you have or have you had any other animals?

Beef Cattle   9.52%

Birds 21.43%

Chickens 20.24%

Dairy Cattle   2.38%

Dog 58.33%

Ducks 17.86%

Fish 29.76%

Geese   9.52%

Goats   5.95%

Horses 14.29%

Insects   4.76%

Pig   5.95%

Reptiles 10.71%

Rodents 16.67%

None   5.95%

49) Have you ever had Mold in your home?

Yes 25.00%

No 48.81%

50) Have you ever lived near a Golf Course or athletic field?

Yes 22.62%

No 51.19%

51) Do you or have you participated in sports on groomed athletic fields?

Yes 32.14%

No 41.67%

52) Do you maintain your own lawn or landscaping?

Yes 50.00%

No 23.81%

With pesticides and herbicides at the forefront of Parkinson's studies it is critical to try to estimate exposure. The exposure rates on golf courses and athletic fields is important to note but home exposure is a significant area that should be studied. People are at much higher risk of this type of exposure at home than in a sports environment. Pesticides and herbicides are readily available for consumer use with little to no regulation after the point of purchase.

One of the biggest downfalls of this is the EPA labeling system. It is far too lax and geared more towards the manufacturer than the consumer. Although consumers might in fact read portions of the labels printed in microscopic text looking for application instructions which are printed in a much larger font than the warnings, it is safe to assume that a majority do not read the dangers listed and do not use them responsibly.

Additionally, many of the chemicals sold without restriction contain harmful binding agents or surfactants. Most of these are simply not regulated and are not required to be listed even though some of them are strongly suspected of causing cancer, neurological problems, and a host of other illnesses. As an example, polyoxyethylene tallow amine is a surfactant used with glyphosate. It is strongly suspected of causing neurological and other disorders, yet it is unregulated by the EPA and is listed as an inert ingredient. This is wrong if not criminal, there's no other way to say it.

The chemical regulation system in the United States is hopelessly broken and the people of America are the one's unwittingly paying the price.

Medical

53) Do you smoke cigarettes?

5-10 per day   3.57%

0-5 per day   4.76%

10-20 per day   5.95%

More than 20 per day 4.76%

Never 38.10%No 13.10%

Smokers are less likely to have Parkinson's. It has been suggested but not proven that nicotine may have neuroprotective effects but to date no studies have proven this. It is also thought that there might be a loss of nicotine receptors in the brain which would diminish the craving for nicotine, this is a more reasonable assumption.

Beyond that, tobacco is a member of the nightshade family which is known to benefit Parkinson's symptoms through liver function via the alkaloids that these plants contain. This is more likely to be the where the benefit lies.

54) Do you have allergies?

Yes 30.95%

No 38.10%

55) Have you ever had a head injury?

Yes 33.33%

No 35.71%

It is known that repeated blows to the head over time can cause Parkinson's like symptoms or Chronic Traumatic Encephalopathy. It is not well understood why this happens. Diagnosis of CTE has improved and it can often be distinguished from idiopathic Parkinson's. It is still under debate as to whether CTE is in fact related to Parkinson's as they are not identical in their presentation.

56) Have you ever had a spinal injury?

Yes 17.86%

No 51.19%

57) Have you had any surgeries?

Yes 55.95%

No 13.10%

58) Have you ever been under Anesthesia?

Yes 64.29%

No 4.76%

59) Do you drink Alcohol?

Never 20.24%

0-5 drinks per week 34.52%

5-10 drinks per week 10.71%

10-20 drinks per week 1.19%

More than 20 drinks per week 2.38%

Alcohol use appears to be fairly moderate. In some cases, it should be considered as a cause. Hepatic Encephalopathy can cause neurological problems and be mistaken for Parkinson's as has been evidenced in some cases.

60) Have you ever used drugs or inhalants for recreational purposes?

Adderall 0.00%

Amphetamines 5.95%

Cialis 1.19%

Cocaine 9.52%

Cough Syrup 4.76%

Diet Pills 2.38%

Formaldehyde (sherm) 0.00%

Gasoline 0.00%

Glue 0.00%

Levitra 1.19%

Heroin 0.00%

LSD 3.57%

Marijuana   21.43%

Morphine 0.00%

MDMA (Ecstasy) 0.00%

Mescaline 2.38%

MPPP 0.00%

None   30.95%

Muscle Relaxers 5.95%

Opium 1.19%

Other Inhalants 1.19%

OxyContin 1.19%

Paint 1.19%

PCP 0.00%

Percocet 1.19%

Psilocybin 0.00%

Ritalin 0.00%

Steroids 0.00%

Valium 2.38%

Viagra 3.57%

Vicodin 1.19%

Drug induced Parkinson's is not common. There are specific types of drugs that are known to cause symptoms. Some are temporary while others are permanent. There is no indication that recreational drug use is a primary cause of Parkinson's disease.

Cases of MPTP intoxication are not common and in fact are somewhat restricted to incidences that occurred with synthetic heroin in the 1980's. MPTP is also not an effective means of inducing Parkinson's because it presents bi-laterally making it of different etiology than idiopathic Parkinson's.

61) "What other medical conditions do you have or have you had in the past? (Diagnosed or Suspected)"

ALS 0.00%

Alzheimer's 0.00%

Anemia 5.95%

Angina 0.00%

Arrhythmia 4.76%

Arthritis   16.67%

Asthma 9.52%

Ataxia 1.19%

Bi-Polar Disorder 3.57%

Bladder Infection   14.29%

Blood Clots 1.19%

Cancer 2.38%

Celiac Disease 0.00%

36

Cervical Myelopathy 0.00%

Circulatory Problems 2.38%

Constipation   26.19%

COPD 2.38%

Edema 4.76%

Epilepsy 0.00%

Dementia 3.57%

Dental Problems   22.62%

Depression   23.81%

Dermatitis 3.57%

Diabetes 3.57%

Diverticulitis 3.57%

Dystonia 5.95%

Eating Disorder 1.19%

Emphysema 0.00%

Encephalitis 0.00%

Eczema 3.57%

Foot Pain   16.67%

Gastro-Intestinal issues   14.29%

Glaucoma 3.57%

Gout 4.76%

Hair Loss   14.29%

Heart Attack 1.19%

Hepatitis 1.19%

Hernia 9.52%

High Blood Pressure   23.81%

HIV 0.00%

Hives 2.38%

HPV 1.19%

HSV1 1.19%

HSV2 0.00%

Hyperreflexia 0.00%

IBS 0.00%

Imbalance 8.33%

Incontinence 7.14%

Kidney Disease 3.57%

Lactose Intolerance 3.57%

Liver Disease 0.00%

Low Blood Pressure 7.14%

Meningitis 0.00%

MSA 0.00%

Multiple Sclerosis 0.00%

Muscle Weakness 3.57%

Neuropathy 5.95%

Obesity 8.33%

OCD 1.19%

Other0.00%

Parkinson's Plus 4.76%

Pancreatitis 0.00%

Pertussis 0.00%

Poor Sense of Smell   28.57%

Poor Sense of Taste   14.29%

Psoriasis 2.38%

Psychiatric Treatment 5.95%

Ptosis 0.00%

Rashes 8.33%

Skin Problems   10.71%

Stomach Ulcer 4.76%

Stroke 2.38%

Thyroid disorder   11.90%

Toxoplasmosis 1.19%

Traumatic Injury 8.33%

Tuberculosis 0.00%

Venereal Disease1.19%

Vertigo 5.95%

Warts   13.10%

Medical history can often provide clues to the cause of other illness. This is not necessarily the case in Parkinson's. Poor sense of smell and constipation have both been attributed to the disease. Why it affects the olfactory senses is not fully understood but it is quite common. Constipation is also extremely common and could be due to lack of serotonin in the gut or poor signaling to the muscles. Depression is seen in a large number of patients and may also be due to serotonin imbalances. Alternatively, depression can also be a psychological aspect of living with the disease.

62) Have you ever been suspected of having Lyme disease?

Yes 5.95%

No 63.10%

63) What was the test result? (If Applicable)

Positive 1.19%

Negative 2.38%

Inconclusive 1.19%

  Not Tested 1.19%

Lyme disease has been frequently been associated with Parkinson's. Most often this is an incorrect assumption and the diagnoses is not made by a neurologist.

Lyme can cause symptoms that are similar to Parkinson's but it is more common to see meningitis, encephalitis, and dementias. Arthritis is common in 60% or more of Lyme patients, especially in the knees. This type of arthritis is not typically seen with Parkinson's.

Late stage Lyme often presents neurologically with bi-lateral involvement which is not typically a sign of idiopathic Parkinson's. In cases that present bi-laterally it is prudent to test for spirochetes such as Lyme and syphilis first as this is a known late stage complication of spirochete infection.

There are enough distinctions between the symptoms of Lyme disease and Parkinson's that a competent neurologist would not confuse the two. There are extremely few documented cases of Lyme being mistaken for Parkinson's. Those that have been were accompanied by other symptoms of Lyme leading up to the neurological involvement.

64) What Medicals tests have you had?

Anemia   8.33%

Bone scan 20.24%

Colonoscopy 32.14%

CT scan 40.48%

DAT scan   7.14%

EEG 20.24%

EKG 39.29%

EMG   7.14%

Endoscopy 11.90%

Genetic Study   9.52%

Lumbar puncture   7.14%

MRI 47.62%

PET scan   5.95%

RPR   1.19%

Sleep Study   9.52%

Standard Blood Tests 51.19%

TCD   1.19%

Urinalysis 39.29%

VDRL 2.38%

VNG   1.19%

X-Ray 52.38%

Other 3.57%

65) Were any of the tests positive or conclusive?

Anemia 3.57%

Bone scan 7.14%

Colonoscopy 9.52%

CT scan   8.33%

DAT scan 3.57%

EEG   1.19%

EMG 1.19%

EKG 2.38%

Endoscopy 3.57%

Genetic Study 1.19%

Lumbar puncture 1.19%

MRI 22.62%

PET scan   2.38%

RBR 1.19%

Sleep Study   2.38%

Standard Blood Tests 10.71%

TCD   1.19%

Urinalysis   7.14%

VDRL   1.19%

VNG   1.19%

EMG   1.19%

X-Ray 13.10%

   Other   9.52%

Testing during a Parkinson's diagnosis can be quite extensive and often reveals other maladies that were previously unknown. MRI's are by far the most common tool when diagnosing Parkinson's but often reveal little of significance. DAT scans showed promise but are typically used to differentiate between Parkinson's and essential tremor. As of yet there is no type of imaging or test that can positively identify the disease making diagnosis difficult.

66) Were any of the following present on an MRI?

Abnormal Parenchymal Signal 1.19%

Basal Ganglia Degeneration 5.95%

Brain Damage 4.76%

Caudus Equinus 0.00%

Chiari 0.00%

Disc Degeneration   20.24%

Flattening of the Pons 0.00%

Foraminal Narrowing 2.38%

Hemorrhage 2.38%

'Hot Cross Buns' sign 0.00%

Hydromyelia 0.00%

Hydrocephalus 0.00%

Ischemia 3.57%

Manganese Intoxication 0.00%

Midline Shift 2.38%

Osteophytosis 2.38%

Pineal Cyst 1.19%

Schmorl's Node 0.00%

Spinal Cord Impingement 3.57%

Spinal Cord Mass 1.19%

Spinal Cord Prominence 0.00%

Stenosis 8.33%

Syringomyelia 0.00%

Tumors 2.38%

Most of what is seen on an MRI will not aid in the diagnosis of Parkinson's, although it can help differentiate between other illnesses, expose tumors, advanced degeneration, and other brain abnormalities. Disc degeneration is quite commonplace and has very little relevance in a Parkinson's diagnosis.

67) Were any of the following abnormal on a CSF exam?

Protein 1.19%

WBC 1.19%

Other 3.57%

There is currently nothing identifiable in a Cerebral Spinal Fluid exam that will confirm a diagnosis of Parkinson's. There has been some progress with identifying protein abnormalities and copper imbalances but nothing clinically relevant as of yet.

68) What motor symptoms are affected?

Chewing   4.76%

Cramping 26.19%

Decreased Arm swing 41.67%

Drooling 23.81%

Dystonia 19.05%

Freezing 27.38%

Grasping 14.29%

Lack of Dexterity 34.52%

Mask like Expression 29.76%

Micrographia (Small handwriting) 30.95%

Postural Instability 26.19%

Reaching   4.76%

Resting Tremor 39.29%

Rigidity 45.24%

Running 13.10%

Sitting   5.95%

Slow Movement 48.81%

Speaking 29.76%

Standing 19.05%

Stooped Posture 23.81%

Tremor 41.67%

Typing 22.62%

Unwanted Accelerations 7.14%

Vision 11.90%

Walking 29.76%

Writing 34.52%

None 1.19%

Diagnosis is most often made by observing and evaluating the symptoms and is often followed with a trial dose of levodopa to confirm it.

Lack of arm swing, slow movement, rigidity, and tremor are the most prominent signs of the disease. Changes in writing, facial expression and lack of dexterity are also strong indicators. There are many different early symptoms that are still being discovered and classified.

69) Are your symptoms Bi-Lateral or Uni-Lateral?

Bi-Lateral (affects both sides) 27.38%

Uni-Lateral (affects one side) 42.86%

One of the criteria of idiopathic Parkinson's is that it usually presents itself as unilateral. Cases that are bilateral are often attributed to Parkinsonism due to a secondary cause. This of course is not always the case but is accepted as a general rule. Secondary Parkinsonism also does not always respond well to levodopa and can have a known cause.

70) Is only your dominant side affected, or was only your dominant side affected at initial onset?

Yes 42.86%

No 26.19%

In recent years studies have indicated that the dominant side is almost disproportionally affected at a ratio of 60% or higher at onset. There is also a different pattern of onset along with initial symptoms. There have been few studies on this and all reach similar conclusions. There certainly must be a reason for this and it should be studied closely until a conclusion is reached.

71) What part of the body is affected?

Back 16.67%

Feet 36.90%

Hands 46.43%

Internal Systems 15.48%

Left Arm 38.10%

Left Leg 38.10%

Neck 26.19%

Right Arm 35.71%

Right Leg 28.57%

It is quite apparent that peripherals are the most affected parts of the body. A point of interest here is that even though peripherals were most affected, they ranked quite low on the pain scale with the exception of the feet.

72) What non motor symptoms do you exhibit?

Breathing Problems   9.52%

Cognitive Problems 23.81%

Constipation 35.71%

Depression 27.38%

Excessive Saliva 19.05%

Fatigue 44.05%

Fear/ Anxiety 29.76%

Impulsiveness 16.67%

Numbness 17.86%

Orthostatic Hypotension   7.14%

Poor sense of smell 40.48%

Poor sense of Taste 19.05%

Sleep Disturbances 41.67%

Swallowing Difficulty 22.62%

Urinary Problems 28.57%

 Weight loss 10.71%

Fatigue and sleep disturbances are often primary complaints in Parkinson's. These may in fact be pre-clinical conditions that are dismissed as stress related or as minor ailments.

A poor sense of smell is commonly associated with Parkinson's, Alzheimer's, and dementias. It may even be an early indicator. Constipation, depression, and urinary problems also common non-motor symptoms.

A common thread with all of these symptoms may in fact be serotonin. It is a precursor to dopamine and also affects many physiological and psychological functions. 80-90% of serotonin is produced in the gastrointestinal tract, the rest is produced in the brain. Additionally, serotonin used by the brain must be produced in the brain. Understanding serotonin, its functions and its production fully could lead to breakthroughs in research for many illnesses.

73) What medications have you been treated with?

Anti-Inflammatory 10.71%

Apokyn   0.00%

Azilect (Rasagiline) 35.71%

Benztropine 0.00%

Carbidopa-Levodopa 52.38%

Entacapone 10.71%

Mirapex 21.43%

Muscle Relaxers 9.52%

Percocet 1.19%

Prednisone 5.95%

Requip (Ropinirole) 20.24%

Selegiline 8.33%

Tolcapone 1.19%

Trihexyphenidyl   1.19%

Other 25.00%

Dopamine replacement is still the most effective treatment for Parkinson's. Carbidopa-Levodopa has been used for more than 40 years. The main side effect of this drug is involuntary movement. It has recently been concluded that Amantadine has some degree of effectiveness at controlling these movements. It is not fully understood why except that it inhibits MAO-A which is typically not associated with Parkinson's.

Dopamine agonists and selective MAO inhibitors are also common drugs used to treat Parkinson's. These classes of drugs can have far ranging and pronounced side effects. Some of the primary concerns with these drugs are psychosis, compulsiveness, a variety of physical side effects and even suicide.

There are a limited number of new drugs being developed for Parkinson's, so this is a trend that is likely to continue for some time.

73) Do you have consistent side effects from Dopamine?

Yes 19.05%

No 33.33%

74) What nondrug treatments have you had?

Acupuncture 13.10%

Ayurvedic Medicine (Holistic) 1.19%

Bone Marrow Transplant   0.00%

Botlinum Toxin A   1.19%

Broad Beans   0.00%

CoQ10 26.19%

DBS   5.95%

Physical Therapy 29.76%

Exercise 58.33%

Massage 26.19%

St. John's Wort   2.38%

Stem Cell Therapy   0.00%

Transfusion   1.19%

Yoga 15.48%

Other   9.52%

75) Were any of them effective?

Acupuncture 5.95%

Anti-Inflammatory 2.38%

Apokyn 0.00%

Ayurvedic Medicine (Holistic) 1.19%

Azilect (Rasagiline) 15.48%

Benztropine 0.00%

Bone Marrow Transplant 0.00%

Botlinum Toxin A 1.19%

Broad Beans 0.00%

Carbidopa-Levodopa 30.95%

CoQ10 2.38%

DBS 5.95%

Physical Therapy 20.24%

Entacapone 4.76%

Exercise 39.29%

Massage 11.90%

Mirapex 13.10%

Muscle Relaxers 3.57%

Percocet 0.00%

Prednisone 0.00%

Requip (Ropinirole) 9.52%

Selegiline 2.38%

St. John's Wort 0.00%

Stem Cell Therapy 0.00%

Tolcapone 1.19%

Transfusion 0.00%

Trihexyphenidyl 0.00%

Yoga 9.52%

None 9.52%

While many treatments are ineffective in part or in full, a few stand out as effective. Dopamine is of course effective. Curiously, exercise and physical therapy outrank all other drug treatments. It is possible that exercise activates the body's detoxification system or somehow stimulates production of neurotransmitters, even if temporary. It is very worthy of investigation.

76) Do you have any of the following Vitamin Deficiencies?

A 1.19%

B 2.38%

B12   11.90%

B6 1.19%

Biotin 0.00%

C 1.19%

Calcium 2.38%

D   20.24%

E 2.38%

Folate 0.00%

Iron 1.19%

K 1.19%

Niacin 0.00%

Riboflavin 0.00%

Unknown   40.48%

Vitamin deficiencies are not extremely common in Parkinson's although there have been associations with low levels of vitamin D. Unfortunately, this is also associated with many other types of illness making it an unreliable measure. Amino acid deficiency and metabolism is probably a better marker as these are the basis for the production of neurotransmitters.

77) Have you had any of the following Immunizations?

Diphtheria 30.95%

Hepatitis A 19.05%

Hepatitis B 15.48%

HPV 1.19%

Influenza 44.05%

Malaria 8.33%

Measles 36.90%

Meningococcal 3.57%

Mumps 32.14%

Pertussis 21.43%

Polio 55.95%

Rabies 4.76%

Rubella 29.76%

Tetanus 60.71%

Varicella 4.76%

Zoster 4.76%

78) What types of Physicians have you seen for this condition?

Cardiologist 11.90%

Chiropractor 10.71%

Dermatologist 4.76%

Endocrinologist 2.38%

Gastrologist 4.76%

General Practitioner/Family Doctor 47.62%

Geneticist 0.00%

Hematologist 0.00%

Hepatologist 0.00%

Mental Health Counselor 7.14%

Naturopath 0.00%

Nephrologist 2.38%

Neurologist 64.29%

Neurophysiologist 5.95%

Neurosurgeon 17.86%

Oncologist 0.00%

Orthopedist 4.76%

Otolaryngologist 0.00%

Pain Specialist/Anesthesiologist 2.38%

Physiatrist 1.19%

Podiatrist 5.95%

Proctologist 0.00%

Psychiatrist 5.95%

Psychologist 5.95%

Pulmonologist 1.19%

Rheumatologist 4.76%

Sleep Doctor 4.76%

Urologist   4.76%

Other 3.57%

79) Do you have or have you had any dental fillings containing Amalgam or Mercury?

Yes 48.81%

No 20.24%

80) Do you still have them?

Yes 36.90%

No 11.90%

Mercury is known to cause neurological problems along with many other types of ailments. The signs of mercury poisoning are actually more pronounced and identifiable than Parkinson's symptoms. The most prominent symptom is tremor. Mercury also has more pronounced effects on cognitive function, mood, and behavior.

Amalgam is often blamed for neurological problems. The limiting factor in this scenario is that it is not understood if amalgam fillings release mercury vapor over time. This is imperative to understand because most cases of mercury poisoning are via the route of inhaled vapor which would not be typically indicative of amalgam fillings. If there is suspicion of dental fillings causing neurological problems they should certainly be removed and any changes noted.

81) How many hours per day on average are you awake?

8-10 hours 4.76%

10-12 hours 4.76%

12-14 hours 14.29%

14-16 hours 26.19%

16-20 hours 19.05%

82) Do you require naps in the daytime to improve your functionality?

Yes 46.43%

No 22.62%

83) Do you have sleep disturbances?

Yes 55.95%

No 13.10%

84) Do you wake in the middle of the night?

Yes 53.57%

No 2.38%

85) Do you wake up around the same time when this occurs?

Yes 33.33%

No 20.24%

86) Are you able to go back to sleep?

Yes 33.33%

No 20.24%

87) What wakes you?

Bladder Issues 30.95%

Breathing difficulty 5.95%

Inability to turn or move 15.48%

Inability to swallow or dry mouth 11.90%

Night Sweats 11.90%

Pain 14.29%

Stiffness 16.67%

Tremor 13.10%

Unknown 16.67%

Sleep disturbances are prevalent in Parkinson's. Why patients wake isn't clearly understood. Waking due to bladder issues once a night is considered normal and can be at least partly discounted as the group that wakes at the same time and is able to return to sleep.

Waking for unknown reasons is as common as physical causes of waking making it a point of interest. Many patients report suddenly being awake during the night as if they had never been asleep. This group has difficulty returning to sleep and often wakes quite early. Most of the other causes of waking are in fact a physical awakening.

There is hypothesis that there may be insufficient melatonin produced in the brain, thus disturbing the sleep cycle. Serotonin is a precursor to melatonin so it is reasonable to associate an imbalance in either of these with sleep disturbances. This does not fully explain the sudden waking.

Cortisol is also an important factor in sleep. Cortisol levels are known to increase in the morning after waking to prepare the body for stress. It is very possible that unknown causes of waking and the inability to return to sleep are due to elevated cortisol levels. Cortisol also has a rate limiting effect on serotonin and in turn melatonin. This could be caused by the body responding to stress while sleeping and releasing cortisol which would lead to suddenly being awake and alert. Perhaps waking in the night is the body mistakenly activating its natural defense mechanisms. There is certainly much more to this but it is a path that should be studied.

Diet

88) Do you eat canned goods?

Broth 30.95%

Condiments 35.71%

Fish 32.14%

Fruit 32.14%

Gravy 14.29%

Jams and Jellies 39.29%

Meat 23.81%

Milk 19.05%

Mushrooms 25.00%

Pasta 17.86%

Peanut Butter 30.95%

Pickled Items 27.38%

Pudding 14.29%

Salad Dressing 32.14%

Sauces 35.71%

Soups 47.62%

Tomato Products46.43%

Vegetables 50.00%

89) Do you eat frozen prepared foods?

Breads 33.33%

Burritos 14.29%

Fish 33.33%

Fruit 21.43%

Ice Cream 53.57%

Juice 19.05%

Meat 40.48%

Pasta 19.05%

Pies 29.76%

Pizza 41.67%

Popsicles 16.67%

Potatoes 29.76%

Seafood 38.10%

Snacks 23.81%

TV Dinners 19.05%

Vegetables 50.00%

90) Do you drink any of the following products?

Alcoholic Mixers   9.52%

Ale 10.71%

Bottled water 48.81%

Breakfast drinks 11.90%

Coffee 50.00%

Cordials   3.57%

Diet soda 25.00%

Energy Drinks   5.95%

Flavored Creamer 13.10%

Hard Liquor 16.67%

Juices 41.67%

Lager Beer 19.05%

Malt   0.00%

Milk 46.43%

Non Dairy Creamer 14.29%

Other flavored beverages 13.10%

Powdered creamer 13.10%

Powdered drink mixes   8.33%

Soda 30.95%

Tap water 51.19%

Tea 42.86%

Weight loss drinks   4.76%

Wheat Beer   8.33%

Wine 38.10%

91) Do you eat any of the following Dairy products?

Aged Cheese 48.81%

Butter 52.38%

Cereals 45.24%

Cheese 59.52%

Chocolate Milk 16.67%

Cottage Cheese 33.33%

Eggs 58.33%

Evaporated Milk 11.90%

Flavored Milk   7.14%

Orange Juice 41.67%

Processed Cheese 34.52%

Pudding 28.57%

Sour Cream 40.48%

Soy Products 14.29%

Tofu 15.48%

Whipped Cream 25.00%

Yogurt 48.81%

92) Do you eat any of the following fast foods?

Chicken 41.67%

Chicken byproducts   8.33%

Desserts 22.62%

Eggs 25.00%

French Fries 46.43%

Hamburger 42.86%

Hot Dogs 21.43%

Onion Rings 27.38%

Other Meat 19.05%

Pastries 25.00%

Pizza 42.86%

Salads 32.14%

Sausage 17.86%

Other 13.10%

93) Do you consume any of the following?

Black Pepper 54.76%

Caffeine 52.38%

Canola Oil 39.29%

Corn Syrup 21.43%

Deli Meats 38.10%

Dried Goods 32.14%

Margarine 40.48%

MRE's 1.19%

MSG 7.14%

Mushrooms (Any Type) 52.38%

Olive Oil 51.19%

Saccharin 7.14%

Salt 47.62%

Soybean Oil 10.71%

Sugar Substitutes 22.62%

Sugars 44.05%

Vegetable Oil 41.67%

Vinegar 46.43%

94) Do you consume any of the following products that may contain Aspartame?

Carbonated soft drinks 34.52%

Chewing gum 22.62%

Confections 11.90%

Dessert mixes 9.52%

Fillings (Fruit etc.) 11.90%

Frozen desserts 16.67%

Gelatins 9.52%

Powdered soft drinks 7.14%

Puddings 11.90%

Sugar-free cough drops 7.14%

Tabletop sweeteners 11.90%

Vitamins 19.05%

Yogurt 29.76%

Other 5.95%

95) Do you eat products that contain Gluten?

Beer 26.19%

Bread 59.52%

Breadcrumbs 30.95%

Broth 20.24%

Cakes 44.05%

Candy 29.76%

Cereal 50.00%

Couscous 21.43%

Crackers 45.24%

Croutons 28.57%

Dressings 32.14%

Durham Wheat 10.71%

Flour Tortillas 34.52%

Fried Foods 32.14%

Graham Flour 10.71%

Gravy 29.76%

Hot-Dogs 26.19%

Imitation Fish 7.14%

Kamut 3.57%

Lunch Meats 30.95%

Matzo   3.57%

Muffins 38.10%

Oats 42.86%

Pasta 50.00%

Pastries 39.29%

Rice 50.00%

Salad Dressing 45.24%

Sauces 39.29%

Semolina 15.48%

Soy Sauce 28.57%

Spelt 10.71%

Triticale   4.76%

Wheat Bran 25.00%

Wheat Germ 16.67%

White Flour 50.00%

96) Do you eat Wild Game or Foul?

Yes 13.10%

No 50.00%

97) Do you eat fish caught fresh from any of the following areas?

Lakes 17.86%

Ocean 48.81%

Other 9.52%

Rivers 14.29%

Sloughs 3.57%

Streams 4.76%

98) Do you eat Shellfish or Crustaceans?

Yes 50.00%

No 13.10%

99) Do you knowingly eat foods grown from genetically modified organisms?

Yes 7.14%

No 55.95%

There are a couple of interesting facts here. This series of questions was created to see if Parkinson's patients have any unusual dietary habits which they do not. It was also structured to assess the intake of foods that are known to contain pesticide residues, chemicals or GMO's which turns it into kind of a trick question. This was quite deliberate.

Only 7% of respondents admitted to knowingly eating foods containing GMO's and 6% knowingly use products containing BPA. This is at the very least educational because a majority of the foods listed contain both GMO's and nearly all can goods are lined with BPA. Nearly 80% of the foods in North America contain GMO's. Plastics often contain BPA or BPS also.

Comparative studies have shown that BPA does in fact leech from canned goods into the food and can be detected in urine at approximately 1000% higher levels than those that do not consume canned goods. BPA has many known health effects as has been banned from infant food containers. It is also suspected of causing a multitude of ailments including but not limited to heart problems, hormone disruption, cancer, and behavioral problems to name a few. The full effect on human health is unknown but animal studies indicate that it is harmful on many levels.

GMO's are a topic of heated debate that is not likely to end anytime soon. Just to be perfectly clear, there is no statistical evidence that connects GMO's to health problems of any kind. Proponents of GMO's are absolutely correct when making this statement. The health effects are genuinely unknown but that doesn't mean that there is not potential for harm to human health.

The problem with GMO's is not necessarily that they are genetically modified or that changes will occur in the DNA of the organism consuming them. The danger lies in the fact that GMO's are designed to be resistant to harmful pesticides and chemicals which are in turn consumed as a part of the food.

Claims that GMO's do not contain pesticide residues are patently false and scientific results are easily manipulated. It is a huge game of smoke and mirrors and a gigantic failure of the FDA and EPA to protect the public through so called regulation.

Chemical manufacturers as well as GMO producers both have the unique ability to provide their own science and statistical data as allowed by the EPA and FDA. This is where the system is intrinsically fails. A majority of studies conducted by corporate producers carefully select substances to be tested. They do not test for chemicals that are considered inert, nor do they test for a full spectrum of chemicals contained in a GMO.

Glyphosate is a good example as previously stated. Glyphosate may not be harmful in and of itself but the surfactants contained in its formulations are strongly suspected of doing damage to enzymes and proteins which certainly has the potential to alter DNA and cause chronic health problems. Glyphosate is one of the most widely used pesticides in the world. It is said to be unavoidable in the environment.

2,4-D is also a widely used chemical on food and other crops. In fact, these two chemicals have been so overused that many weeds have become naturally resistant to them. This will continue to happen no matter what formulations are used.

2,4-D is a non-selective herbicide that was a component of Agent Orange in the Vietnam war. Serious health effects were noted including Parkinson's type syndromes. It was 'determined' that the combination of 2,4-D and 2,4,5-T led to the production of harmful dioxins when overheated. Ultimately 2,4,5-T was banned and the continued use of 2,4-D was allowed, in fact it was expanded. As it turns out, the 2,4,5-T combination was not the sole cause of dioxin contamination.

Within the last decade the EPA estimated that up to 25% of 2,4-D formulations were contaminated with dioxins. Dioxins are persistent in the environment and know to accumulate in tissue over a lifetime. A majority of dioxin exposure occurs through the food we eat. That is directly from the EPA. In 2014 the EPA vastly increased the allowable amount of glyphosate and 2,4-D to be released into the environment. Additionally, they also approved a combined formulation of the two for use on food crops. This may in fact be the proverbial nail in the coffin as damage caused by these chemicals cannot be reversed.

These regulations must be changed if we are to continue to survive. Humans as well as animals are being systematically poisoned on a daily basis. Unfortunately, this is due to vast amounts of money funneled from corporations into government to create these regulatory loopholes allowing the widespread use of these toxic chemicals.

Consumption of fish is also a potential route to chemical exposure. Certainly, ocean fish and shellfish are likely to be contaminated with mercury and other toxic substances. Lake and stream fish are also likely to contain phosphates and other land based chemicals that have contaminated the water. Without widespread testing it cannot be known how broad this exposure is. One thing for certain is that if we continue to devastate our oceans and inland waters, we will find ourselves living in a barren wasteland. We cannot continue this path of environmental destruction and not expect to suffer severe consequences.

Chemicals

100) Do you knowingly use products Containing BPA?

Yes   5.95%

No 54.76%

101) Do you use products containing 2,4-D?

Yes   9.52%

No 51.19%

102) Do you use any of the following chemicals?

Acetone 19.05%

Aerosol Insect Killer 26.19%

Alkaloids   3.57%

Ammonia 17.86%

Antifreeze 20.24%

Beauty Products 27.38%

Bleach 41.67%

Borax 10.71%

Boric Acid   7.14%

Brake Fluid 14.29%

Briquettes 10.71%

Butane 14.29%

Car Wax 20.24%

Carwash Soap 17.86%

Caulking 21.43%

Contac Solution 10.71%

Dishwasher Drying Agents 23.81%

Drain Cleaner 20.24%

Dyes of any type 13.10%

Fabric Softener 35.71%

Fertilizer 30.95%

Fluoride Toothpaste 48.81%

Furniture Polish 29.76%

Glue/Contact Cement 29.76%

Hairspray 25.00%

Hand Soap 50.00%

Hydrogen Peroxide 34.52%

Kerosene 15.48%

Laundry Soap 44.05%

Lead   1.19%

Lighter Fluid 11.90%

Lotions 35.71%

Mecoprop   2.38%

Molybdenum   3.57%

Non-stick Cooking Sprays 36.90%

Oven Cleaner 23.81%

Powdered Cleanser 23.81%

Propane 17.86%

Rubbing Alcohol 28.57%

Salt 50.00%

Sodium Hydroxide   7.14%

Solvents 20.24%

Spray Paint 26.19%

Spray Starch 10.71%

Sulfur   4.76%

Tarnish Remover 10.71%

Toilet Cleaner 38.10%

Turpentine 15.48%

Weed Killer 32.14%

Window Cleaner 39.29%

Yard Insect Killer 30.95%

103) Do you use products containing Teflon?

Yes 44.05%

No 15.48%

104) Do you always wash new clothing before you wear it?

Yes 17.86%

No 41.67%

Chemicals have been used for centuries. Most early use and production of chemicals was probably an unintentional byproduct of the use of fire and in metallurgy followed by different types of alchemy.

Modern day chemicals began to develop in the late 19th century and have become a staple of modern society.

Chemicals have become inescapable and are found in nearly every part of the world and society.

Most chemicals are petroleum based derivatives and are highly toxic, many with unknown effects on health. Solvents are widely used and are most often synthesized, petroleum based or chlorine based. Those are just the most common types. As our knowledge of chemistry grows, so does our ability to create even more toxic chemicals. Unfortunately, the production, invention and approval of chemicals rapidly outpaces the development and approval of new drugs. Ironically, many of these much needed drugs must be developed to combat illness caused by the chemicals we use.

The toxic load on our bodies is greater now than it has ever been. We use chemicals on a daily basis without fully understanding what they are. There is a tremendous lack of education in regard to household and industrial use alike.

The results contained in the chemical section are probably consistent with the use of the average person without Parkinson's. Multiply that by 5 to 7 billion and that will give an indication of how heavily saturated our planet has become with chemicals. The difference with Parkinson's is probably lifetime exposure or toxic load combined with genetic susceptibility.

Parkinson's could also be caused by a combination of specific chemicals which essentially creates the perfect storm and causes permanent genetic damage. With the tremendous lack of oversight and regulation we may never know. Research simply cannot keep up with this path of destruction that we are on.

As an individual, the best thing that you can do is drastically limit your use of chemicals to protect your health. This means using mild soap and water to clean rather than toxic chemicals, avoiding canned and packaged good, driving less, and growing your own food if you have the means. It will only benefit you. This is especially important if you have Parkinson's or some other chronic illness. This should be a growing trend and become the norm rather than the exception. It will take time which is quickly escaping us. We each need to do our part and remember that battleships don't turn on a dime and we need to turn this one around. Awareness may be the most important aspect of this battle we will be facing to save ourselves and it starts with you.

Work Exposure

105) Have you worked in any of the following Industries?

Agriculture 15.48%

Automotive 7.14%

Automotive (Manufacturing) 1.19%

Computer (Manufacturing) 2.38%

Construction 14.29%

Cosmetics (Any Area) 3.57%

Chemical 3.57%

Electrical (Any Area) 5.95%

Electronics (Manufacturing) 2.38%

Fishing 3.57%

Food 16.67%

Fur 0.00%

Garment 3.57%

Health Care 9.52%

HVAC 1.19%

Law Enforcement 3.57%

Manufacturing 5.95%

Metalworking 3.57%

Military 5.95%

Mining 2.38%

Petroleum 1.19%

Pharmaceutical (Manufacturing) 1.19%

Plumbing 3.57%

Pulp/Paper 1.19%

Shipping 2.38%

Textile 1.19%

Timber 1.19%

Tobacco (Production) 0.00%

Toy (Manufacturing) 0.00%

Transportation 3.57%

Welding 3.57%

Other 27.38%

106) Have you ever had contact with 'Agent Orange'?

Yes 3.57%

No 55.95%

107) Have you ever come in contact with Napalm?

Yes 1.19%

No 58.33%

Working is one of the more common routes of exposure to chemicals. Not surprisingly construction and agriculture show the highest percentage in this data set. This is probably due to the fact that there is open chemical exposure in these industries and the size of them. There really hasn't been a direct correlation with Parkinson's outside of agricultural jobs and pesticide use. The higher percentage in the food industry is likely an anomaly due strictly to the size of the industry. Of course, Agent Orange exposure in the military is being blamed for many of the cases of Parkinson's in veterans and it's probably accurate. Interestingly most studies indicate that the majority of Parkinson's patients have maintained indoor desk jobs. What could that possibly indicate?

Medications

108) What medications have you taken in the past?

ACE Inhibitors 5.95%

Acetaminophen 40.48%

Antacids 35.71%

Anti-Inflammatory 35.71%

Antibacterial 23.81%

Antibiotics 53.57%

Antidepressants 29.76%

Antiviral 4.76%

Apokyn 0.00%

Atrazine 1.19%

Azilect (Rasagiline) 29.76%

Entacapone 10.71%

Benztropine 0.00%

Beta Blockers 9.52%

Carbidopa-Levodopa 40.48%

Codeine 28.57%

Dextromethorphan   9.52%

Haloperidol   0.00%

Ibuprofen 46.43%

Lipid regulators 9.52%

MAO Inhibitors 13.10%

Metoclopramide   0.00%

Mirapex 21.43%

Muscle Relaxers 23.81%

Naprosyn 11.90%

Narcotic Analgesics 10.71%

Percocet 17.86%

Phenothiazine   0.00%

Prednisone 13.10%

Prozac   9.52%

Pseudoephedrine   9.52%

Requip 15.48%

Sedatives/Tranquilizers 13.10%

Selegiline   5.95%

Tolcapone   2.38%

Trihexphenidyl   1.19%

Zoloft   5.95%

Other 14.29%

109) What medications do you currently take?

ACE Inhibitors   3.57%

Acetaminophen 10.71%

Antacids 10.71%

Anti-Inflammatory   9.52%

Antibacterial   1.19%

Antibiotics   0.00%

Antidepressants 11.90%

Antiviral   1.19%

Apokyn   0.00%

Atrazine   0.00%

Azilect (Rasagiline) 23.81%

Entacapone   7.14%

Benztropine   0.00%

Beta Blockers   4.76%

Carbidopa-Levodopa 39.29%

Codeine   1.19%

Dextromethorphan   0.00%

Haloperidol   0.00%

Ibuprofen 27.38%

Lipid regulators 5.95%

MAO Inhibitors   2.38%

Metoclopramide   0.00%

Mirapex 13.10%

Muscle Relaxers   3.57%

Naprosyn   3.57%

Narcotic Analgesics   1.19%

Percocet   0.00%

Phenothiazine   0.00%

Prednisone   0.00%

Prozac   1.19%

Pseudoephedrine   1.19%

Requip   7.14%

Sedatives/Tranquilizers   5.95%

Selegiline   3.57%

Tolcapone   1.19%

Trihexphenidyl   1.19%

Zoloft   1.19%

Other 14.29%

110) What Supplements do you take?

Amino Acids 1.19%

Antioxidants 13.10%

Arginine 0.00%

Calcium 10.71%

Choline   0.00%

CoQ10 14.29%

Creatine 3.57%

Energy (Including herbal) 2.38%

Fat Loss 1.19%

Lysine 1.19%

Magnesium 5.95%

Multi Vitamin 22.62%

Muscle Builders 0.00%

Niacin   1.19%

Omegas 10.71%

Other Herbal Supplements 5.95%

Potassium 2.38%

Protein 1.19%

Vitamin A   2.38%

Vitamin B12 22.62%

Vitamin B6   8.33%

Vitamin C   7.14%

Vitamin D 23.81%

Whey Protein   2.38%

Other 19.05%

The use of both over the counter and prescription drugs combined has grown incredibly. According to the CDC, patients were prescribed drugs 75% of the time or more in both physician and hospital visits. In 2010 2.6 billion prescriptions were ordered from office visits alone. Supplements were not far behind and adult use has grown to around 60%.

Obviously in conditions such as Parkinson's drugs are an absolute necessity. Some are more effective than others. The benefits of certain drugs must outweigh the risk and many times they don't. Prescription drugs are more tightly regulated due to side effects and potential for addiction. They are still rampantly over prescribed. Drugs should be taken at the minimum level needed to be therapeutic, nothing more.

Although there are around 35 different drugs used for Parkinson's disease, only a limited number are used.

Carbidopa-Levodopa is bar far the most used and most effective. The drawback as with any drug is the development of involuntary movements with prolonged use. Amantadine appears to be somewhat effective at controlling these movements for a few years. This of course treads on the dangerous ground of using one drug to control the detrimental side effects of another. This is fairly common unfortunately and a clear indication that human biology is not well understood. This is still the safest path of treatment in Parkinson's if the patient is responsive to it.

I'm not going to go into great detail about the drugs. Most of us know what they are and what they do. Azilect and other MAO inhibitors are also commonly prescribed for Parkinson's. I recommend not taking them if at all possible. They are often not effective and can have disturbing side effects. I say that from personal experience. Take what you need to be functional and avoid drugs with heavy side effects.

Over the counter drugs are ripe for abuse due to the widespread availability. Pain killers such as ibuprofen and acetaminophen are commonly used and should probably be limited to the minimum. Acetaminophen has been shown to cause severe liver damage resulting in a restructuring of the guidelines for taking it. This should have occurred nearly 40 years ago when it first became evident. Long term ibuprofen use increases the risk of heart attack and stroke. Just because it is sold over the counter does not mean that it is 100% safe.

Another problem not often mentioned about supplements and over the counter medications that is important to Parkinson's patients are the effects of the buffers. Cellulose and Alum are commonly used as buffers and binders for pills. What does this mean for the Parkinson's patient? In short it can translate into constipation which is the last thing a person with Parkinson's needs.

There are many other effects from over the counter medications that are undesirable, some may have interactions with prescription medications. Always research drugs or supplements of any kind before taking them, you may actually feel better without some of them.

Supplements do not appear to have any beneficial effect on Parkinson's. It is best to obtain vitamins from food through proper diet. This has actually proven to be quite effective for many. Our bodies are simply not designed to obtain nutrients by taking pills. Taking supplements isn't as direct as it seems. If you are taking vitamin B-12 alone for example, it is highly likely that you are not fully absorbing it if at all. In order for the body to absorb B-12 the body also needs B-6 and B-9 (folate) to properly absorb it. This is the case with many supplements including amino acids. If you take supplements it is probably best to stick to liquids if possible, perhaps even just a multi-vitamin. There is no need to overload on these products or even take them if they are not recommended by your doctor.

Fresh and unprocessed foods are the most desirable because they are organic matter that contains a variety of vitamins, minerals, and amino acids that our bodies can effectively process. Mother Nature has a recipe and it works.

In Conclusion

I felt it was important to share the data from the Parkinson's Database Survey© to provide others with data and information about Parkinson's. I believe it is important to researchers as well as patients. It at the very least provides an opportunity for patients to look at data collected from others suffering from the same illness. It gives people some opportunity to make comparisons and perhaps even make some simple changes for their own benefit.

I've spent countless hours studying this disease and learned a great deal about it and how to live with it. It's a struggle sometimes but its life as I know it now and I'm ok with it.

I know I've added a lot of commentary with this data set. It is based on my opinions and also based on the research and the survey results. The survey will continue to be available online indefinitely and probably be amended or followed by more specific surveys that are based on the results.

There is a lot of research being done on Parkinson's. Some of it is relevant and quite frankly some of it is absurd. There honestly hasn't been a great deal of breakthrough research in recent years. Certainly, there are studies funded and conducted but the core features and understanding of Parkinson's has changed little in the last decade.

My experience has been that it is difficult to find a great deal of information on Parkinson's in one place. I often read what appear to be new studies only to discover that they are nothing more than combined reviews of earlier research. It is fairly obvious that scientists are for lack of a better word 'stumped'.

There has to be a tipping of the scales with this disease at some point. Perhaps it's time to go about research in a different manner. Patients are the most valuable source of information when it comes to these types of illnesses. Actively listening to them would open many doors.

There could also be some revisions in FDA policy when it comes to drug approval. It is such a time consuming and laborious process that it literally takes years to bring a new drug to market. Other countries don't appear to have these same problems getting drugs or treatments to patients. If we didn't rely so heavily on animal testing, we might not have so many failures. Yes, we are biologically similar but at the same time we are different. The government needs to revise its overly restrictive policies on both clinical trials and funding. There is a lot of good research out there that isn't being given a chance because it doesn't meet the criteria for government grants. This needs to change now not later.

One of the more bothersome discoveries I made was the disposition of the National Neurological Surveillance Act. This bill was introduced twice and would create a national registry for Parkinson's disease and make it a reportable illness. Both times it was presented it was referred to committee and didn't even receive a vote. The cost was one ten thousandth of one percent of the annual budget. It is almost unbelievable that this happened not once but twice. It shows what a low priority our politicians place on Parkinson's disease.

Interestingly enough there is a national ALS registry as well as a national MS registry. The MS registry provided valuable data and research quickly moved forward. This should be the case for Parkinson's. There are a few registries for Parkinson's maintained by Universities and some states but they are not interconnected nor are they required. With today's technology it really is a simple matter. I believe that it can be done easily with minimal cost but it must have some kind of backing. It does not have to be intrusive into people's lives or violate their right to privacy. I think that is clearly demonstrated by the fact that I was able to accomplish this with the database.

In closing, if you are suffering from Parkinson's, be vigilant and do everything you can to better your life. Share what you know and discover with others. Have faith that a cure will be discovered. Take part in any way you can to help change this broken system, there is strength in numbers.

Most importantly:

Be well,

Steven